C000203256

The Inspired Ketogenic Cookbook for Beginners

Delicious and Healthy Ketogenic Recipes to Boost Your Day and Improve Your Lifestyle

Lauren Loose

Contents

Ketogenic white rice

Total time: 65 minutes

Ingredients :

1 cup of rice

1 cup of diced tomatoes

1 ¼ cups of diced peppers

Extra virgin olive oil ½ cup

½ cup of boiled ground beef

1/8 cup of diced green onions

1/8 cup of sliced spring onions

Salt

Adobo seasoning

Directions

Put 3-4 cups of water in a large saucepan and bring to boil

Put in your rice when it starts to boil and put in a table spoon of salt

After 16-20 minutes, the rice should be ready. If you aren't quite sure, you can fish it for a grain or three to taste

There should still be lots of water in the pot and so, you should strain it out. Straining the water drains out some of the starch which means you reduce the carbs. You can use a strainer with tiny holes.

Place your strained rice in a pot and cover.

Preheat your saucepan

Pour in your extra virgin oil and let it heat very slightly

Pour in your diced green onions. Fry for 15 seconds. While frying, stir it so it doesn't burn

Put in your spring onions and fry for another 15 seconds. Remember to stir.

Put in your pepper and stir for half a minute

Put in your tomatoes and stir.

Stir together for 5-7 minutes

Put in your boiled ground beef

Put in a teaspoon of salt

Put in a teaspoon of Adobo seasoning

Stir together for 5-8 minutes

Place your boiled rice in a serving dish.

Spread your sauce over the rice.

Enjoy hot or warm

Steamed veggies and prawn with coconut milk

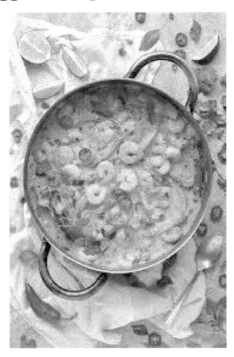

Total time: 45 minutes

Ingredients :

1 pound of fresh shrimps

4 tablespoons of extra virgin olive oil

1 egg

1/8 cup of coconut milk

½ cup almond flour

¼ cup water

1/8 of cup grated cheddar cheese

1/8 cup of diced carrot

1/8 of cup diced onion

1/8 of cup chopped leek

Directions

Peel prawns, remove heads and set aside

Crack an mix an egg in a bowl

Mix water and almond flour with water

Pour in half of the egg

Mix with a spoon

Use the mixture to make omelets

Take your peeled prawns and put them in a food processor

Process till smooth

Preheat a skillet

Pour in 1 ½ spoons of the olive oil

Put in onion and sauté. Stir fry till it is golden brown

Add the leak and carrot and stir for ten seconds

Pour in coconut milk

Stir till the milk disappears

Put the cooked veggies, prawns, and remaining half egg into the bowl

Mix well

Put an omelet on a plate and put a tablespoon of the prawn mix

Fold the omelet like an envelope

Repeat with the rest of the omelets

Preheat a saucepan and then pour the remaining olive oil into it.

When the oil is a bit hot, put the prawn envelopes in the saucepan

Cook for 2 minutes on each side till golden brown

Serve warm

Mediterranean pork chops

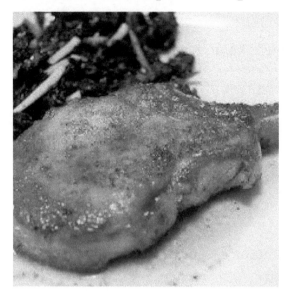

Total time: 45 minutes

Ingredients :

8 boneless pork loin chops

1 teaspoon of black pepper

1 teaspoon of kosher salt

7 minced garlic cloves

2 tablespoon of chopped and fresh rosemary

Directions

Mix garlic and rosemary in a bowl

Place pork chops in a bowl. Sprinkle pepper and salt

Rub in the salt and pepper

Rub in garlic and rosemary

Place pork chops in roasting pan at 425 degrees F. Do this for ten minutes

Reduce the temperature of the oven to 350 F degrees and continue roasting for about 20-25 minutes

Serve warm

Ketogenic Sloppy Joes

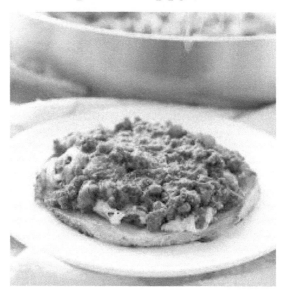

Total time: 45 minutes

Ingredients :

1 ¼ cup almond flour (for the bread)

5 tbsp. ground psyllium husk powder (for the bread)

1 tsp. sea salt (for the bread)

2 tsp. baking powder (for the bread)

2 tsp. cider vinegar (for the bread)

1 ¼ cups boiling water (for the bread)

3 egg whites (for the bread)

2 tbsp. olive oil (for the meat sauce)

1 ½ lbs. ground beef (for the meat sauce)

1 yellow onion (for the meat sauce)

4 garlic clover (for the meat sauce)

14 oz. crushed tomatoes (for the meat sauce)

1 tbsp. chili powder (for the meat sauce)

1 tbsp. Dijon powder (for the meat sauce)

1 tbsp. red wine vinegar (for the meat sauce)

4 tbsp. tomato paste (for the meat sauce)

2 tsp. salt (for the meat sauce)

¼ tsp ground black pepper (for the meat sauce)

½ cup mayonnaise as toppings

6 oz. shredded cheese as toppings

Directions:

We're going to start by cooking the bread. First, preheat the 350 degrees Fahrenheit and then mix all the dry ingredients in a bowl.

Add some vinegar, egg whites, and boiling water in the bowl. Whisk thoroughly for 30 seconds or use a hand mixer to speed up the process. You'd want a consistency that's a lot like play-doh

Form the dough into 5 or 8 pieces of bread. Layer then on the lowest oven rack and cook for 55 to 60 minutes.

In the meantime, you'll be cooking the meat sauce. Grab a pan and cook the onion and garlic until you get that fragrant smell.

Add the ground beef and cook the meat thoroughly. Once done, add the other ingredients and cook

Allow it to simmer for 10 minutes in low heat. Add other seasonings to taste.

Low Carb Crack Slaw Egg Roll in a Bowl Recipe

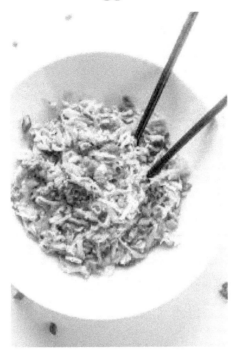

Total time: 20 minutes

Ingredients :

1 lb. ground beef

4 cups shredded coleslaw mix

1 tbsp. avocado oil

1 tsp. sea salt

¼ tsp. black pepper

4 cloves garlic, minced

3 tbsp. fresh ginger, grated

¼ cup coconut aminos

2 tsp. toasted sesame oil

¼ cup green onions

Directions:

Start by heating the avocado oil in a large pan using a medium-high heat. Put in the garlic and cook for a little bit until you get that fragrant smell.

Add the ground beef and cook until it gets brownish. This should take about 10 minutes to finish. Season with salt and black pepper.

Once cooked, you can lower the heat and add the coleslaw mix and the coconut aminos. Stir to cook for 5 minutes or until the coleslaw gets tender.

Remove and put in the green onions and the toasted sesame oil.

Low Carb Beef Stir Fry

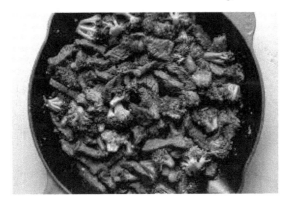

Total time: 25 minutes

Ingredients :

½ cup zucchini, spiral them into noodles about 6-inches each

¼ cup organic broccoli florets

1 bunch baby bok choy, stem chopped

2 tbsp. avocado oil

2 tsp. coconut aminos

1 small know of ginger, peeled and cut

8 oz. skirt steak, thinly sliced into strips

Directions:

Heat the pan and add 1 tablespoon of oil. Sear the steak on it on high heat. This should only take around 2 minutes per side.

Reduce the heat to medium and put in the broccoli, ginger, ghee, and coconut aminos. Cook for a minute, stirring as often as possible.

Add in the bok choy and cook for another minute

Finally, put the zucchini into the mix and cook. Note that zucchini noodles cook quickly so you'd want to pay close attention to this.

One Pan Pesto Chicken and Veggies

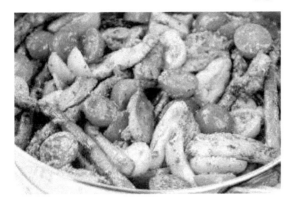

Total time: 35 minutes

Ingredients :

2 tbsp. olive oil

1 cup cherry diced tomatoes

¼ cup basil pesto

1/3 cup sun-dried tomatoes, chopped and drained

1 pound chicken thigh, bones and skinless, sliced into strips

1 pound asparagus, cut in half with the ends trimmed

Directions:

Start by heating up a large skillet. Put two tablespoons of olive oil and sliced chicken on medium heat. Season with salt and add ½ cup of the sun-dried tomatoes.

Cook for a few minutes until the chicken is cooked thoroughly. Spoon out the chicken and tomatoes and put them in a separate container.

Don't wash the skillet just yet. You'll be using the oil there later.

Next, put the asparagus in the skillet and pour in the pesto. Turn the heat on medium and add the remaining sun-dried tomatoes. Cook the asparagus for 5 to 10 minutes. Put it on a separate plate when done.

Put the chicken back in the skillet and pour in pesto. Stir under medium heat for 2 minutes. You only need to reheat the chicken during this so when done, you can serve it together with the asparagus.

Crispy Peanut Tofu and Cauliflower Rice Stir-Fry

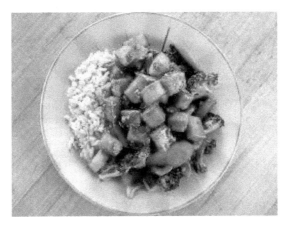

Total time: 1 hour 35 minutes

Ingredients :

12 oz. tofu, extra-firm

1 tbsp. toasted sesame oil

2 cloves minced garlic

1 small cauliflower head

1 ½ tbsp. toasted sesame oil (sauce)

½ tsp. chili garlic sauce (sauce)

2 ½ tbsp. peanut butter (sauce)

¼ cup low sodium soy sauce (sauce)

½ cup light brown sugar (sauce)

Directions:

Start by draining the tofu for 90 minutes before getting the meal ready. You can dry the tofu quickly by rolling it on an absorbent towel and putting something heavy on top. This will create a gentle pressure on the tofu to drain out the water.

Preheat the oven to 400 degrees Fahrenheit. While the oven heats up, cube the tofu and prepare your baking sheet.

Bake for 25 minutes and allow it to cool.

Combine the sauce ingredients and whisk it thoroughly until you get that well-blended texture. You can add more ingredients, depending on your personal preferences with taste.

Put the tofu in the sauce and stir it quickly to coat the tofu thoroughly. Leave it there for 15 minutes or more for a thorough marinate.

While the tofu marinates, shred the cauliflower into rice- size bits. You can also try buying cauliflower rice from the store to save yourself this step. If you're doing this manually, use a fine grater or a food processor.

Grab a skillet and put it on medium heat. Start cooking the veggies on a bit of sesame oil and just a little bit of soy sauce. Set it aside.

Grab the tofu and put it on the pan. Stir the tofu frequently until it gets that nice golden brown color. Don't worry if some of the tofu sticks to the pan – it will do that sometimes. Set aside.

Steam your cauliflower rice for 5 to 8 minutes. Add some sauce and stir thoroughly.

Now it's time to add up the ingredients together. Put the cauliflower rice with the veggies and tofu. Serve and enjoy. You can reheat this if there are leftovers, but try not to leave it in the fridge for long.

Simple Ketogenic Fried Chicken

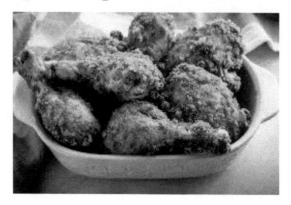

Total time: 45 minutes

Ingredients :

4 boneless and skinless chicken thighs

Frying oil

2 large eggs

2 tbsp. heavy whipping cream

2/3 cup grated parmesan cheese (breading)

2/3 cup blanched almond flour (breading)

1 tsp. salt (breading)

½ tsp. black pepper (breading)

½ tsp. cayenne (breading)

½ tsp. paprika (breading)

Directions:

Grab a bowl and put together the eggs and heavy cream. Beat them together until perfectly mixed.

Grab another bowl, this time combining all the breading ingredients and mix well. Set it aside for now.

Cut the chicken thigh into 3 even pieces. Make sure they're not wet by patting the moist area with a paper towel. This will help prevent the oil splashes when you start frying them.

So now you have the chicken and 2 bowls. One bowl contains the egg wash and the other contains the breading. Dip the chicken in the bread first before dipping it in the egg wash and then finally, dipping it in the breading again. Make sure it's completely covered.

Put 2 inches worth of oil in a pot and heat it up until it reaches around 350 degrees Fahrenheit or when it starts to become steamy. When this happens, try to gradually lower the heat so you can maintain that temperature. This is important since a perfectly heated oil will help create really crunchy chicken.

Put the coated chicken in your hot oil. Do this gently with a pair of tongs, making sure there are no splashes of any kind. Frying time should take around 5 minutes or until the coating becomes deep brown in color.

Prepare some paper towels and put the cooked chicken on it. This will help remove any excess oil.

Try not to overcrowd the pan so all of them will cook beautifully. Serve while still crispy for best results.

Ketogenic Butter Chicken

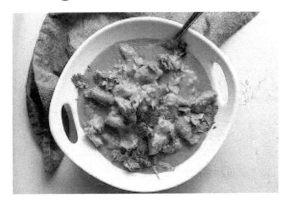

Total time: 35 minutes

Ingredients :

1.5 lb. chicken breast

1 tbsp. coconut oil

2 tbsp. garam masala

3 tsp. grated fresh ginger

3 tsp. minced garlic

4 oz. plain yogurt

2 tbsp. butter (for sauce)

1 tbsp. ground coriander (for sauce)

½ cup heavy cream (for sauce)

½ tbsp. garam masala (for sauce)

2 tsp. fresh ginger, grated (for sauce)

2 tsp. minced garlic (for sauce)

2 tsp. cumin (for sauce)

1 tsp. chili powder (for sauce)

1 onion (for sauce)

14.5 oz. crushed tomatoes (for sauce)

Salt to taste (for sauce)

Directions:

Start by cutting the chicken into pieces measuring around 2 inches each. Place it in a large bowl and add 2 tablespoons of garam masala, 1 teaspoon of minced garlic, and 1 teaspoon of grated ginger. Stir slowly and add the yogurt. Make sure that mix is evenly distributed before putting a lid on the container and chilling it in the fridge for 30 minutes.

For the sauce, grab a blender and put in the ginger, garlic, onion, tomatoes, and spices. Blend until smooth.

Leave the blended sauce aside and grab a skillet. Using medium heat, remove the chicken from the fridge and cook, allowing it to brown on both sides.

Once cooked, pour in the sauce and allow it to simmer for 5 more minutes

Finally, put in the cream and ghee, still using medium heat. Add some salt for taste and serve!

Ketogenic Shrimp Scampi Recipe

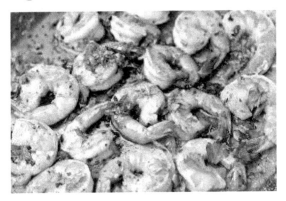

Total time: 35 minutes

Ingredients :

2 summer squash

1 pound shrimp, deveined

2 tbsp. butter unsalted

2 tbsp. lemon juice

2 tbsp. chopped parsley

¼ cup chicken broth

1/8 tsp. red chili flakes

1 clove minced garlic

Salt and pepper to taste

Directions:

Start by cutting the summer squash into noodle-like shapes. You can use a spiralizer to get this done or perhaps use a fork to scrap the surface.

Spread the noodles on top of paper towards and sprinkle them with salt. Set aside for 30 minutes.

Blot the excess water with a paper towel.

In a frying pan, melt butter over medium heat and fry the garlic until you get that fragrant smell. Add some chicken broth, red chili flakes, and lemon juice.

Once it boils, add the shrimp and allow it to cook. Reduce the heat once the shrimp turns pink.

Add more salt and pepper to taste before adding the summer squash noodles and parsley to the mix. Make sure all the ingredients are well-coated by the sauce. Serve.

Ketogenic Lasagna

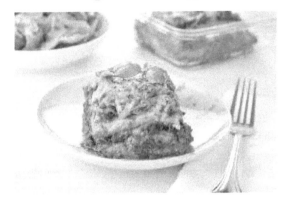

Total time: 1 hour 35 minutes

Ingredients :

8 oz. block of cream cheese

3 large eggs

Kosher salt

Ground black pepper

2 cups of shredded mozzarella

½ cup of freshly grated parmesan

Pinch crushed red pepper flakes

Chopped parsley for garnish

¾ cup marinara (for the sauce)

1 tbsp. tomato paste (for the sauce)

1 lb. ground beef (for the sauce)

½ cup of freshly grated parmesan (for the sauce)

1.5 cup of shredded mozzarella (for the sauce)

1 tbsp. of extra virgin olive oil (for the sauce)

1 tsp. dried oregano (for the sauce)

3 cloves minced garlic (for the sauce)

½ cup chopped onion (for the sauce)

16 oz. ricotta (for the sauce)

Directions:

Start by preheating the oven to 350 degrees and preparing the baking tray by lining it with parchment and cooking spray.

Grab a microwave-safe bowl and throw in the cream cheese, mozzarella, and parmesan, melting them together for a few seconds in the microwave. Mix them in thoroughly before adding the eggs and blending the whole thing together. Add a pinch of salt and pepper for seasoning.

Spread the mixture on a baking sheet and bake for 15 to 20 minutes.

While baking, grab a skillet and using medium heat, coat the surface with oil. Put in the onion and allow them to cook for 5 minutes before adding the garlic. Once you get that fragrant smell, wait 60 more seconds before adding the tomato paste onto the mixture. Make sure to stir all the items around until the onion and garlic are well-coated.

Add the ground beef in the skillet and cook the mixture, breaking up the meat until it's no longer pink in appearance. Add salt and pepper to taste. Cook it for a few more minutes before setting it aside and allowing it to cool. There should be a bit of fluid remaining in the skillet – try to drain that out of the meat before proceeding with the next step.

Turn on the stove again, keeping the medium heat constant. Add some marinara sauce and season with pepper, red pepper flakes, and ground pepper. Stir around to evenly distribute the flavor.

By this time, your noodles should be ready from the oven. Take them out and start cutting them in half width-wise and then cut them again into 3 pieces.

Start layering! Use an 8 inch baking pan for this, placing 2 noodles at the bottom of the dish first and layer as you wish. Alternate the parmesan and mozzarella shreds depending on your personal preferences.

Bake until the cheese melts and the sauce bubbles out. Should take about 30 minutes.

Garnish and serve.

Creamy Tuscan Garlic Chicken

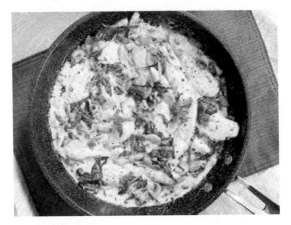

Total time: 30 minutes

Ingredients :

1.5 pounds boneless and skinless chicken breast, thinly sliced

½ cup chicken broth

½ cup parmesan cheese

½ cup sun dried tomatoes

1 cup heavy cream

1 cup chopped spinach

2 tbsp. olive oil

1 tsp. garlic powder

1 tsp. Italian seasoning

Directions:

Grab a large skillet and cook the chicken using olive oil using medium heat. Do this for 5 minutes for each side or until they're thoroughly cooked. Set it aside in a plate.

Using the same skillet, combine the heavy cream, garlic powder, Italian seasoning, parmesan cheese, and chicken broth. Expose it to medium heat and just whisk away until the mixture thickens.

Add the sundried tomatoes and spinach and let it simmer until the spinach wilts.

Add the chicken back and serve.

Cole Slaw Ketogenic Wrap

Preparation Time: 15 minutes

Cooking Time: 0 minutes

Servings: 2

Ingredients:

For the coleslaw

3 cups sliced thin Red Cabbage.

0.5 cups diced Green Onions.

0.75 cups Mayo

2 teaspoons Apple Cider Vinegar

0.25 teaspoon Salt

For the wraps and additional filling

16 pieces, stems removed Collard Green.

1 pound, cooked & chilled Ground Meat of choice

0.33 cup Alfalfa Sprouts

Directions:

Mix slaw items with a spoon in a large-sized bowl until everything is well-coated.

Place a collard green on a plate and scoop a tablespoon or two of coleslaw on the edge of the leaf. Top it with a scoop of meat and sprouts.

Roll and tuck the sides to keep the filling from spilling.

Once you assemble the wrap, put in your toothpicks in a way that holds the wrap together until you are ready to beat it. Just repeat this with the leftover leaves.

NOTE: we can store these for 4-5 days, and 4 wraps make for 1 serving.

Nutrition:

Net carbs: 4g

Fiber: 2g

Fat: 42g

Protein: 2g

Calories: 409

Ketogenic Chicken Club
Lettuce Wrap

Preparation Time: 15 minutes

Cooking Time: 15 minutes

Servings: 1

Ingredients:

1 head of iceberg lettuce with the core and outer leaves removed.

1 tbsp. of mayonnaise

6 slices or organic chicken or turkey breast

Bacon (2 cooked strips, halved)

Tomato (just 2 slices)

Directions:

Line your working surface with a large slice of parchment paper.

Layer 6-8 large leaves of lettuce in the center of the paper to make a base of around 9-10 inches.

Spread the mayo in the center and lay with chicken or turkey, bacon, and tomato.

Starting with the end closest to you, roll the wrap like a jelly roll with the parchment paper as your guide. Keep it tight and halfway through, roll tuck in the ends of the wrap.

When it is completely wrapped, roll the rest of the parchment paper around it, and use a knife to cut it in half.

NOTE: This recipe makes one serve, but the wraps will keep for 3-4 days so you can increase the recipe to have some prepped for lunch through the week.

Nutrition:

Net carbs: 4g

Fiber: 2g

Fat: 78g

Protein: 28g

Calories: 837

Ketogenic Broccoli Salad

Preparation Time: 10 minutes

Cooking Time: 0 minutes

Servings: 4-6

Ingredients:

For your salad

2 medium-sized heads, florets chunked Broccoli.

2 cups shredded well Red Cabbage.

0.5 cups roasted Sliced Almonds.

1 stalk sliced Green Onions.

0.5 cups Raisins

For your orange almond dressing

0.33 cup Orange Juice

0.25 cup Almond Butter

2 tablespoons Coconut Aminos

1; small-sized, chopped finely Shallot.

Half-teaspoon Salt

Directions:

Use a food processor to pulse together salt, shallot, amino, nut butter, and OJ. Make sure it is perfectly smooth.

Use a medium-sized bowl to combine other ingredients. Toss it with dressing and serve.

NOTE: This recipe is around 4-6 serving and can keep for up to 5 days.

Nutrition:

Net carbs: 13g

Fiber: 0g

Fat: 94g

Protein: 22g

Calories: 1022

Caribbean Jerk Shrimp with Cauliflower Rice

Preparation Time: 30 minutes

Cooking Time: 40 minutes

Servings: 8

Ingredients:

For the dish

10 ounces, deveined & peeled Large-sized Shrimp

2 tablespoons EVOO

2 tablespoon) Red Wine Vinegar

2 tablespoons Orange Juice

1 tablespoon packed) Brown Sugar.

1 tablespoon Soy Sauce

2 stalks chopped Green Onions.

1 small-sized, seeded & chopped Jalapenos.

Jerk Seasoning:

a half-teaspoon Powdered Garlic

a half-teaspoon Powdered Onion

0.25 teaspoon Thyme

a half-teaspoon Paprika

0.125 teaspoons Allspice

0.125 teaspoons Nutmeg

0.25 teaspoon Powdered Cayenne

0.125 teaspoons Salt

Lime Wedges

For the cauliflower rice

1 tablespoon EVOO

1; small-sized, chopped Green Pepper.

1; small-sized, seeded & chopped Jalapeno.

1 cup chopped Pineapple.

4 cups Cauliflower Rice

1 teaspoon Powdered Garlic

0.25 teaspoon Salt

0.25 teaspoon Pepper

0.125 teaspoons Cinnamon

0.25 cup Orange Juice

1–15 ounce can, drained Red Kidney Beans

2 tablespoons, chopped fresh herb Cilantro

Directions:

Prepare the marinade first by combining all items from the list. Stir in the shrimp; marinade for only 45 minutes.

Prepare the rice now by combining everything to the skillet from that list. Wait to add cilantro until everything else is warmed. After about 10 minutes, add this herb in.

Now, make the skewers by putting the shrimp on the sticks and grill them outside or on the stovetop. They will probably need 5 minutes per side.

Boil the leftover marinade in a small pot over medium-high temperature. After 1 minute, simmer at low heat for only 10 minutes. Spoon this glaze onto the shrimp. Add rice to the bottom of the prep containers, finishing with adding the shrimp and lime wedges.

Nutrition:

Net carbs: 46g

Fiber: 0g

Fat: 12g

Protein: 30g

Calories: 400 kcal

Ketogenic Sheet Pan Chicken and Rainbow Veggies

Preparation Time: 15 minutes

Cooking Time: 25 minutes

Servings: 4

Ingredients:

Nonstick spray

Chicken Breasts (1 pound, boneless & skinless)

Sesame Oil (1 tablespoon)

Soy Sauce (2 tablespoons)

Honey (2 tablespoons)

Red Pepper (2; medium-sized, sliced)

Yellow Pepper (2; medium-sized, sliced)

Carrots (3; medium-sized, sliced)

Broccoli (half-a-head cut up)

2 Red Onions (medium-size and sliced)

EVOO (2 tablespoons)

Pepper & salt (to taste)

Parsley (0.25 cup, fresh herb, chopped)

Directions:

Spray your baking sheet with cooking spray and bring the oven to a temperature of 400-degrees.

Put the chicken in the middle of the sheet. Separately, combine the oil and the soy sauce. Brush the mix over the chicken.

Like the image above shows, separate your veggies across the plate. Sprinkle with oil and then toss them gently to ensure they are coated. Finally, spice up with pepper & salt.

Set tray into the oven and cook for around 25 minutes until all is tender and done throughout.

After taking out of the oven, garnish using parsley. Divide everything between those prep containers paired with your favorite greens.

NOTE: This recipe makes 4 servings and will keep for 4-5 days.

Nutrition:

Net carbs: 9g

Fiber: 0g

Fat: 30g

Protein: 30g

Calories: 437kcal

Skinny Bang Bang
Zucchini Noodles

Preparation Time: 15 minutes

Cooking Time: 15 minutes

Servings: 4

Ingredients:

For the noodles

4 medium zucchini spiralized

1 tbsp. olive oil

For the sauce

Plain Greek Yogurt (0.25 cup + 2 tablespoons)

Mayo (0.25 cup + 2 tablespoons)

Thai Sweet Chili Sauce (0.25 cup + 2 tablespoons)

Honey (1.5 teaspoons)

Sriracha (1.5 teaspoons)

Lime Juice (2 teaspoons)

Directions:

If you are using any meats for this dish such as chicken or shrimp, cook them first then set aside. Pour the oil into a large-sized skillet at medium temperature. After the oil heats through, stir in the spiraled zucchini noodles. Cook the "noodles" until tender yet still crispy. Remove from the heat, drain, and set at rest for at least 10 minutes.

Combine sauce items together into a large-sized until perfectly smooth. Give it a taste and adjust as needed. Divide into 4 small containers. Mix your noodles with any meats you cooked and add to meal prep containers.

When you are ready to eat it, heat the noodles, drain any excess water, and mix in sauce.

NOTE: This recipe will keep for 3 days.

Nutrition:

Net carbs: 18g

Fiber: 0g

Fat: 1g

Protein: 9g

Calories: 161g

Ketogenic Caesar Salad

Preparation Time: 15 minutes

Cooking Time: 0 minutes

Servings: 4

Ingredients:

Mayonnaise (1.5 cups)

Apple Cider Vinegar / ACV (3 tablespoons)

Dijon Mustard (1 teaspoon)

Anchovy Filets (4)

Romaine Heart Leaves (24 of them)

Pork Rinds (4 ounces, chopped)

Parmesan (for garnish)

Directions:

Place the mayo with ACV, mustard, and anchovies into a blender and process until smooth and dressing like.

Prepare romaine leaves and pour out dressing across them evenly.

Top with pork rinds and enjoy.

NOTE: Keep the dressing in separate small containers until you are ready to eat a salad. This recipe should keep for 4-5 days.

Nutrition:

Net carbs: 4g

Fiber: 3g

Fat: 86g

Protein: 47g

Calories: 993kcal

Ketogenic Buffalo Chicken Empanadas

Preparation Time: 20 minutes

Cooking Time: 30 minutes

Servings: 6

Ingredients:

For the empanada dough

1 ½ cups of mozzarella cheese

3 oz. of cream cheese

1 whisked egg

2 cups of almond flour

For the buffalo chicken filling

2 cups of cooked shredded chicken

Butter (2 tablespoons, melted)

Hot Sauce (0.33 cup)

Directions:

Bring the oven to a temperature of 425-degrees.

Put the cheese & creamed cheese into a microwave-safe dish. Microwave at 1-minute intervals until completely combined.

Stir the flour and egg into the dish until it is well-combined. Add any additional flour for consistency - until it stops sticking to your fingers.

With another medium-sized bowl, combine the chicken with sauce and set aside.

Cover a flat surface with plastic wrap or parchment paper and sprinkle with almond flour. Spray a rolling pin to avoid sticking and use it to press the dough flat. Make circle shapes out of this dough with a lid, a cup, or a cookie cutter. For excess dough, roll back up and repeat the process.

Portion out a spoonful of filling into these dough circles but keep them only on one half. Fold the other half over to close into half-moon shapes. Press on the edges to seal them.

Lay on a lightly greased cooking sheet and bake for around 9 minutes until perfectly brown.

NOTE: This recipe prepares 6 servings and can keep for 4-5 days.

Nutrition:

Net carbs: 20g

Fiber: 0g

Fat: 96g

Protein: 74g

Calories: 1217kcal

Pepperoni and Cheddar Stromboli

Preparation Time: 15 minutes

Cooking Time: 20 minutes

Servings: 3

Ingredients:

Mozzarella Cheese (1.25 cups)

Almond Flour (0.25 cup)

Coconut Flour (3 tablespoons)

Italian Seasoning (1 teaspoon)

Egg (1 large-sized; whisked)

Deli Ham (6 ounces; sliced)

Pepperoni (2 ounces; sliced)

Cheddar Cheese (4 ounces; sliced)

Butter (1 tablespoon, melted)

Salad Greens (6 cups)

Directions:

First things first, bring the oven to a temperature of 400 degrees and prepare a baking tray with some parchment paper.

Use the microwave to melt the mozzarella until it becomes easy to stir.

Mix flours & Italian seasoning in a separate small-sized bowl.

Dump in the melty cheese and stir together with pepper and salt to taste.

Stir in the egg and process the dough with your hands. Pour it onto that prepared baking tray.

Roll out the dough with your hands or a pin. Cut slits that mark out 4 equal rectangles.

Put the ham and cheese onto the dough, then brush with butter and close, putting the seal end down. Bake for around 17 minutes until well-browned. Slice up and serve.

NOTE: This makes 3 servings and will keep for 2-3 days. It is best served with a small salad.

Nutrition:

Net carbs: 20g

Fiber: 0g

Fat: 13g

Protein: 11g

Roasted Cornish Hen

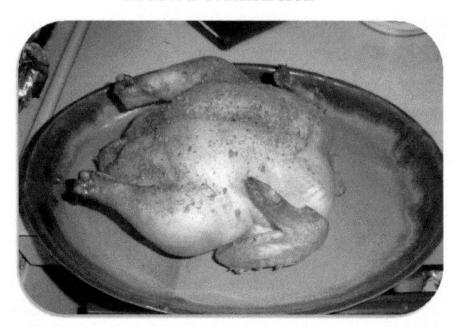

Preparation time: 15 minutes

Cooking time: 1 hour

Servings: 8

Ingredients:

1 tablespoon dried basil, crushed.

2 tablespoons lemon pepper

1 tablespoon poultry seasoning

Salt, as required.

4 (1½-pound) Cornish game hens rinsed and dried completely.

2 tablespoons olive oil

1 yellow onion, chopped.

1 celery stalk, chopped.

1 green bell pepper seeded and chopped.

Directions:

Preheat your oven to 375ºF. Arrange lightly greased racks in 2 large roasting pans.

In a bowl, mix well basil, lemon pepper, poultry seasoning, and salt.

Coat each hen with oil and then, rub evenly with the seasoning mixture.

In a next bowl, mix the onion, celery, and bell pepper.

Stuff the cavity of each hen loosely with veggie mixture.

Arrange the hens into prepared roasting pans, keeping plenty of space between them.

Roast for about 60 minutes or until the juices run clear.

Remove the hens from oven and place onto a cutting board.

With a foil piece, cover each hen loosely for about 10 minutes before carving.

Cut into desired size pieces and serve.

Nutrition:

Calories 714

Net Carbs 2.8 g

Total Fat 52.2 g

Saturated Fat 0.5g

Cholesterol 349 mg

Sodium 235 mg

Total Carbs 3.8 g

Fiber 1 g

Sugar 1.4 g

Protein 58.2 g

Butter Chicken

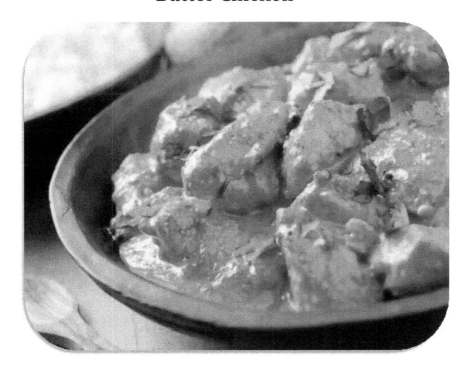

Preparation time: 15 minutes

Cooking time: 28 minutes

Servings: 5

Ingredients:

3 tablespoons unsalted butter

1 medium yellow onion, chopped.

2 garlic cloves, minced.

1 teaspoon fresh ginger, minced.

1½ pounds grass-fed chicken breasts, cut into ¾-inch
   chunks.

2 tomatoes chopped finely.

1 tablespoon garam masala

1 teaspoon red chili powder

1 teaspoon ground cumi n

 Salt and ground black pepper, as required.

1 cup heavy cream

2 tablespoons fresh cilantro, chopped.

Directions:

Melt butter in a large wok over medium-high heat and sauté the onions for about 5–6 minutes.

Now, add in ginger and garlic and sauté for about 1 minute.

Add the tomatoes and cook for about 2–3 minutes, crushing with the back of spoon.

Stir in the chicken spices, salt, and black pepper, and cook for about 6–8 minutes or until desired doneness of the chicken.

Stir in the heavy cream and cook for about 8–10 more minutes, stirring occasionally.

Garnish with fresh cilantro and serve hot.

Nutrition:

Calories 507

Net Carbs 4 g

Total Fat 33.4 g

Saturated Fat 18.6 g

Cholesterol 203 mg

Sodium 211 mg

Total Carbs 5.5 g

Fiber 1.5 g

Sugar 2.3 g

Protein 40.5 g

Chicken & Broccoli Casserole

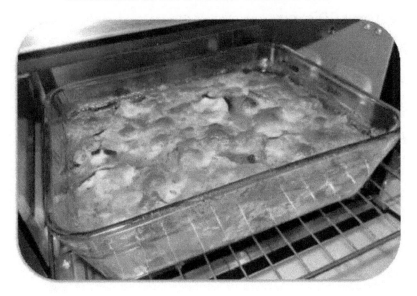

Preparation time: 15 minutes

Cooking time: 35 minutes

Servings: 6

Ingredients

2 tablespoons butter

¼ cup cooked bacon, crumbled.

2½ cups cheddar cheese, shredded and divided.

4 ounces cream cheese, softened.

¼ cup heavy whipping cream

½ pack ranch seasoning mix

2/3 cup homemade chicken broth

1½ cups small broccoli florets

2 cups cooked grass-fed chicken breast, shredded.

Directions:

Preheat your oven to 350ºF.

Arrange a rack in the upper portion of the oven.

For chicken mixture: In a large wok, melt the butter over low heat.

Add the bacon, ½ cup of cheddar cheese, cream cheese, heavy whipping cream, ranch seasoning, and broth, and with a wire whisk, beat until well combined.

Cook for about 5 minutes, stirring frequently.

Meanwhile, in a microwave-safe dish, place the broccoli and microwave until desired tenderness is achieved.

In the wok, add the chicken and broccoli and mix until well combined.

Remove from the heat and transfer the mixture into a casserole dish.

Top the chicken mixture with the remaining cheddar cheese.

Bake for about 25 minutes.

Now, set the oven to broiler.

Broil the chicken mixture for about 2–3 minutes or until cheese is bubbly.

Serve hot.

Nutrition:

Calories 449

Net Carbs 2.3 g

Total Fat 33.5 g

Saturated Fat 20.1 g

Cholesterol 133 mg

Sodium 1001 mg

Total Carbs 2.9 g

Fiber 0.6 g

Sugar 0.8 g

Protein 31.3 g

Turkey Chili

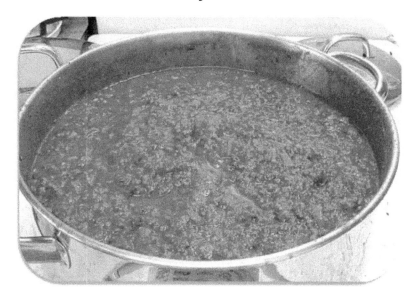

Preparation time: 15 minutes

Cooking time: 2¼ hours

Servings: 8

Ingredients

2 tablespoons olive oil

1 small yellow onion, chopped.

1 green bell pepper seeded and chopped.

4 garlic cloves, minced.

1 jalapeño pepper, chopped.

1 teaspoon dried thyme, crushed.

2 tablespoons red chili powder

1 tablespoon ground cumin

2 pounds lean ground turkey

2 cups fresh tomatoes chopped finely.

2 ounces sugar-free tomato paste

2 cups homemade chicken broth

1 cup water

Salt and ground black pepper, as required.

1 cup cheddar cheese, shredded.

Directions:

In a large Dutch oven, heat oil over medium heat and sauté the onion and bell pepper for about 5–7 minutes.

Add the garlic, jalapeño pepper, thyme, and spices and sauté for about 1 minute.

Add the turkey and cook for about 4–5 minutes.

Stir in the tomatoes, tomato paste, and cacao powder, and cook for about 2 minutes.

Add in the broth and water and bring to a boil.

Now, reduce the heat to low and simmer, covered for about 2 hours.

Add in salt and black pepper and remove from the heat.

Top with cheddar cheese and serve hot.

Nutrition:

Calories 234

Net Carbs 4.8 g

Total Fat 12.6 g

Saturated Fat 3.2 g

Cholesterol 81 mg

Sodium 328 mg

Total Carbs 6.9 g

Fiber 2.1 g

Sugar 3.2 g

Protein 24.9 g

Beef Curry

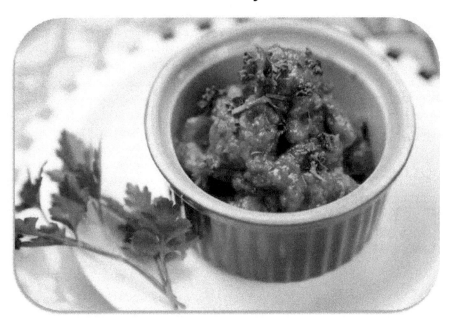

Preparation time: 10 minutes

Cooking time: 3¼ hours

Servings: 8

Ingredients

2 tablespoons butter

2 tomatoes chopped finely.

2 tablespoons curry powder

2½ cups unsweetened coconut milk

½ cup homemade chicken broth

2½ pounds grass-fed beef chuck roast, cubed into 1-inch size.

Salt and ground black pepper, as required.

¼ cup fresh cilantro, chopped.

Directions:

Melt butter in a large pan over low heat and cook the tomatoes and curry powder for about 3–4 minutes, crushing the tomatoes with the back of spoon.

Stir in the coconut milk, and broth, and bring to a gentle simmer, stirring occasionally.

Simmer for about 4–5 minutes.

Stir in beef and bring to a boil over medium heat.

Adjust the heat to low and cook, covered for about 2½ hours, stirring occasionally.

Remove from heat and with a slotted spoon, transfer the beef into a bowl.

Set the pan of curry aside for about 10 minutes.

With a slotted spoon, remove the fats from top of curry.

Return the pan over medium heat.

Stir in the cooked beef and bring to a gentle simmer.

Adjust the heat to low and cook, uncovered for about 30 minutes or until desired thickness.

Stir in salt and black pepper and remove from the heat.

Garnish with fresh cilantro and serve hot.

Nutrition:

Calories 666

Net Carbs 3.2 g

Total Fat 53 g

Saturated Fat 27 g

Cholesterol 154 mg

Sodium 204 mg

Total Carbs 4.1 g

Fiber 0.9 g

Sugar 2.8 g

Protein 38.8 g

Shepherd's Pie

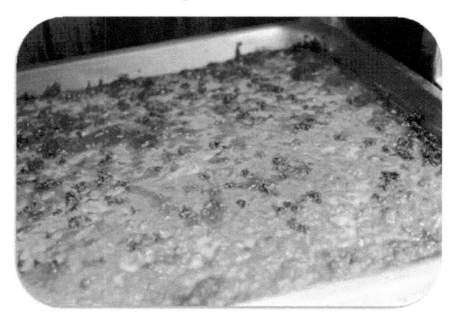

Preparation time: 20 minutes

Cooking time: 50 minutes

Servings: 6

Ingredients

¼ cup olive oil

1-pound grass-fed ground beef

½ cup celery, chopped.

¼ cup yellow onion, chopped.

3 garlic cloves, minced.

1 cup tomatoes, chopped.

2 (12-ounce) packages riced cauliflower cooked and well drained.

1 cup cheddar cheese, shredded.

¼ cup Parmesan cheese, shredded.

1 cup heavy cream

1 teaspoon dried thyme

Directions:

Preheat your oven to 350ºF.

Heat oil in a large nonstick wok over medium heat and cook the ground beef, celery, onions, and garlic for about 8–10 minutes.

Remove from the heat and drain the excess grease.

Immediately stir in the tomatoes.

Transfer mixture into a 10x7-inch casserole dish evenly.

In a food processor, add the cauliflower, cheeses, cream, and thyme, and pulse until a mashed potatoes-like mixture is formed.

Spread the cauliflower mixture over the meat in the casserole dish evenly.

Bake for about 35–40 minutes.

Remove casserole dish from oven and let it cool slightly before serving.

Cut into desired sized pieces and serve.

Nutrition:

Calories 404

Net Carbs 5.7 g

Total Fat 30.5 g

Saturated Fat 13.4 g

Cholesterol 100 mg

Sodium 274 mg

Total Carbs 9.2 g

Fiber 3.5 g

Sugar 4 g

Protein 24.5 g

Meatballs Curry

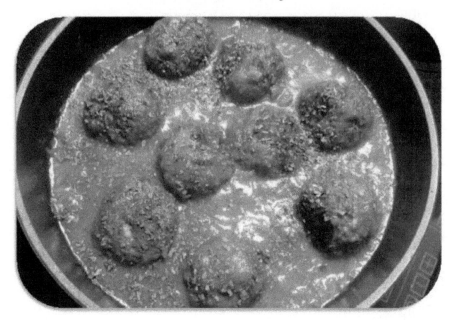

Preparation time: 15 minutes

Cooking time: 25 minutes

Servings: 6

Ingredients

Meatballs

1-pound lean ground pork

2 organic eggs, beaten.

3 tablespoons yellow onion finely chopped.

¼ cup fresh parsley leaves, chopped.

¼ teaspoon fresh ginger, minced.

2 garlic cloves, minced.

1 jalapeño pepper seeded and finely chopped.

1 teaspoon granulated erythritol

1 teaspoon curry powder

3 tablespoons olive oil

Curry

1 yellow onion, chopped.

Salt, as required.

2 garlic cloves, minced.

¼ teaspoon fresh ginger, minced.

1 tablespoon curry powder

1 (14-ounce) can unsweetened coconut milk

Ground black pepper, as required.

¼ cup fresh parsley, minced.

Directions:

For meatballs: Place all the ingredients (except oil) in a large bowl and mix until well combined.

Make small-sized balls from the mixture.

Heat the oil in a large wok over medium heat and cook meatballs for about 3–5 minutes or until golden-brown from all sides.

Transfer the meatballs into a bowl.

For curry: In the same wok, add onion and a pinch of salt, and sauté for about 4–5 minutes.

Add the garlic and ginger, and sauté for about 1 minute.

Add the curry powder and sauté for about 1–2 minutes.

Add coconut milk and meatballs and bring to a gentle simmer.

Adjust the heat to low and simmer, covered for about 10–12 minutes.

Season with salt and black pepper and remove from the heat.

Top with parsley and serve.

Nutrition:

Calories 350

Net Carbs 4.2 g

Total Fat 29.1 g

Saturated Fat 9.7 g

Cholesterol 55 mg

Sodium 73 mg

Total Carbs 5.2 g

Fiber 1 g

Sugar 2.7 g

Protein 16.2 g

Pork with Veggies

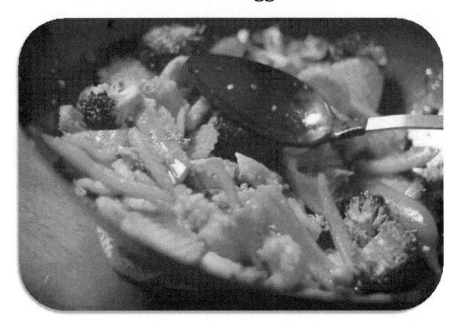

Preparation time: 15 minutes

Cooking time: 15 minutes

Servings: 5

Ingredients

1-pound pork loin cut into thin strips.

2 tablespoons olive oil, divided.

1 teaspoon garlic, minced.

1 teaspoon fresh ginger, minced.

2 tablespoons low-sodium soy sauce

1 tablespoon fresh lemon juice

1 teaspoon sesame oil

1 tablespoon granulated erythritol

1 teaspoon arrowroot starch

10 ounces broccoli florets

1 carrot peeled and sliced.

1 large red bell pepper seeded and cut into strips.

2 scallions cut into 2-inch pieces.

Directions:

In a bowl, mix well pork strips, ½ tablespoon of olive oil, garlic, and ginger.

For sauce: Add the soy sauce, lemon juice, sesame oil, Swerve, and arrowroot starch in a small bowl and mix well.

Heat the remaining olive oil in a large nonstick wok over high heat and sear the pork strips for about 3–4 minutes or until cooked through.

With a slotted spoon, transfer the pork into a bowl.

In the same wok, add the carrot and cook for about 2–3 minutes.

Add the broccoli, bell pepper, and scallion, and cook, covered for about 1–2 minutes.

Stir the cooked pork, sauce, and stir fry, and cook for about 3–5 minutes or until desired doneness, stirring occasionally.

Remove from the heat and serve.

Nutrition:

Calories 315

Net Carbs 5.7 g

Total Fat 19.4 g

Saturated Fat 5.7 g

Cholesterol 73 mg

Sodium 438 mg

Total Carbs 8.3 g

Fiber 2.6 g

Sugar 3 g

Protein g Classic
Pork Tenderloin

Preparation Time: 15 minutes

Cooking Time: 35 minutes

Servings: 4

Ingredients:

8 bacon slices

2 lb. pork tenderloin

1 tsp. dried oregano, crushed.

1 tsp. dried basil, crushed.

1 tbsp. garlic powder

1 tsp. seasoned salt

3 tbsp. butter

Directions:

Preheat the oven to 400 degrees F.

Heat a large ovenproof skillet over medium-high heat and cook the bacon for about 6-7 minutes.

Transfer the bacon onto a paper towel lined plate to drain.

Then, wrap the pork tenderloin with bacon slices and secure with toothpicks.

With a sharp knife, slice the tenderloin between each bacon slice to make a medallion.

In a bowl, mix the dried herbs, garlic powder and seasoned salt.

Now, coat the medallion with herb mixture.

With a paper towel, wipe out the skillet.

In the same skillet, melt the butter over medium-high heat and cook the pork medallion for about 4 minutes per side.

Now, transfer the skillet into the oven.

Roast for about 17-20 minutes.

Remove the wok from oven and let it cool slightly before cutting.

Cut the tenderloin into desired size slices and serve.

Nutrition:

Calories per serving: 471.

Carbohydrates: 1g.

Protein: 53.5g.

Fat: 26.6g.

Sugar: 0.1g.

Sodium: 1100mg.

Fiber: 0.2g

Signature Italian Pork Dish

Preparation Time: 15 minutes

Cooking Time: 15 minutes

Servings: 6

Ingredients:

2 lb. pork tenderloins cut into 1½-inch pieces.

¼ C. almond flour

1 tsp. garlic salt

Freshly ground black pepper, to taste.

2 tbsp. butter

½ C. homemade chicken broth

1/3 C. balsamic vinegar

1 tbsp. capers

2 tsp. fresh lemon zest grated finely.

Directions:

In a large bowl, add the pork pieces, flour, garlic salt and black pepper and toss to coat well.

Remove pork pieces from bowl and shake off excess flour mixture.

In a large skillet, melt the butter over medium-high heat and cook the pork pieces for about 2-3 minutes per side.

Add broth and vinegar and bring to a gentle boil.

Reduce the heat to medium and simmer for about 3-4 minutes.

With a slotted spoon, transfer the pork pieces onto a plate.

In the same skillet, add the capers and lemon zest and simmer for about 3-5 minutes or until desired thickness of sauce.

Pour sauce over pork pieces and serve.

Nutrition:

Calories per serving: 373.

Carbohydrates: 1.8g.

Protein: 46.7g.

Fat: 18.6g.

Sugar: 0.4g.

Sodium: 231mg.

Fiber: 0.7g

Flavor Packed Pork Loin

Preparation Time: 15 minutes

Cooking Time: 1 hour

Servings: 6

Ingredients:

1/3 C. low-sodium soy sauce

¼ C. fresh lemon juice

2 tsp. fresh lemon zest, grated.

1 tbsp. fresh thyme finely chopped.

2 tbsp. fresh ginger, grated.

2 garlic cloves chopped finely.

2 tbsp. Erythritol

Freshly ground black pepper, to taste.

½ tsp. cayenne pepper

2 lb. boneless pork loin

Directions:

For pork marinade: in a large baking dish, add all the ingredients except pork loin and mix until well combined.

Add the pork loin and coat with the marinade generously.

Refrigerate for about 24 hours.

Preheat the oven to 400 degrees F.

Remove the pork loin from marinade and arrange into a baking dish.

Cover the baking dish and bake for about 1 hour.

Remove from the oven and place the pork loin onto a cutting board.

With a piece of foil, cover each loin for at least 10 minutes before slicing.

With a sharp knife, cut the pork loin into desired size slices and serve.

Nutrition:

Calories per serving: 230.

Carbohydrates: 3.2g.

Protein: 40.8g.

Fat: 5.6g.

Sugar: 1.2g.

Sodium: 871mg.

Fiber: 0.6g

Spiced Pork Tenderloin

Preparation Time: 15 minutes

Cooking Time: 18 minutes

Servings: 6

Ingredients:

2 tsp. fresh rosemary, minced.

2 tsp. fennel seeds

2 tsp. coriander seeds

2 tsp. caraway seeds

1 tsp. cumin seeds

1 bay leaf

Salt and freshly ground black pepper, to taste.

2 tbsp. fresh dill, chopped.

2 (1-lb.) pork tenderloins, trimmed.

Directions:

For spice rub: in a spice grinder, add the seeds and bay leaf and grind until finely powdered.

Add the salt and black pepper and mix.

In a small bowl, reserve 2 tbsp. of spice rub.

In another small bowl, mix the remaining spice rub, and dill.

Place 1 tenderloin over a piece of plastic wrap.

With a sharp knife, slice through the meat to within ½-inch of the opposite side.

Now, open the tenderloin like a book.

Cover with another plastic wrap and with a meat pounder, gently pound into ½-inch thickness.

Repeat with the remaining tenderloin.

Remove the plastic wrap and spread half of the dill mixture over the center of each tenderloin.

Roll each tenderloin like a cylinder.

With a kitchen string, tightly tie each roll at several places.

Rub each roll with the reserved spice rub generously.

With 1 plastic wrap, wrap each roll and refrigerate for at least 4-6 hours.

Preheat the grill to medium-high heat. Grease the grill grate.

Remove the plastic wrap from tenderloins.

Place tenderloins onto the grill and cook for about 14-18 minutes, flipping occasionally.

Remove from the grill and place tenderloins onto a cutting board and with a piece of foil, cover each tenderloin for at least 5-10 minutes before slicing.

With a sharp knife, cut the tenderloins into desired size slices and serve.

Nutrition:

Calories per serving: 313.

Carbohydrates: 1.4g.

Protein: 45.7g.

Fat: 12.6g.

Sugar: 0g.

Sodium: 127mg.

Fiber: 0.7g

Sticky Pork Ribs

Preparation Time: 15 minutes

Cooking Time: 2 hours 34 minutes

Servings: 9

Ingredients:

¼ C. Erythritol

1 tbsp. garlic powder

1 tbsp. paprika

½ tsp. red chili powder

4 lb. pork ribs, membrane removed.

Salt and freshly ground black pepper, to taste.

1½ tsp. liquid smoke

1½ C. sugar-free BBQ sauce

Directions:

Preheat the oven to 300 degrees F. Line a large baking sheet with 2 layers of foil, shiny side out.

In a bowl, add the Erythritol, garlic powder, paprika and chili powder and mix well.

Season the ribs with salt and black pepper and then, coat with the liquid smoke.

Now, rub the ribs with the Erythritol mixture.

Arrange the ribs onto the prepared baking sheet, meaty side down.

Arrange 2 layers of foil on top of ribs and then, roll and crimp edges tightly.

Bake for about 2-2½ hours or until desired doneness.

Remove the baking sheet from oven and place the ribs onto a cutting board.

Now, set the oven to broiler.

With a sharp knife, cut the ribs into serving sized portions and evenly coat with the barbecue sauce.

Arrange the ribs onto a broiler pan, bony side up.

Broil for about 1-2 minutes per side.

Remove from the oven and serve hot.

Nutrition:

Calories per serving: 530.

Carbohydrates: 2.8g.

Protein: 60.4g.

Fat: 40.3g.

Sugar: 0.4g.

Sodium: 306mg.

Fiber: 0.5g

Valentine's Day Dinner

Preparation Time: 15 minutes

Cooking Time: 35 minutes

Servings: 4

Ingredients:

1 tbsp. olive oil

4 large boneless rib pork chops

1 tsp. salt

1 C. cremini mushrooms chopped roughly.

3 tbsp. yellow onion chopped finely.

2 tbsp. fresh rosemary, chopped.

1/3 C. homemade chicken broth

1 tbsp. Dijon mustard

1 tbsp. unsalted butter

2/3 C. heavy cream

2 tbsp. sour cream

Directions:

Heat the oil in a large skillet over medium heat and sear the chops with the salt for about 3-4 minutes or until browned completely.

With a slotted spoon, transfer the pork chops onto a plate and set aside.

In the same skillet, add the mushrooms, onion and rosemary and sauté for about 3 minutes.

Stir in the cooked chops, broth and bring to a boil.

Reduce the heat to low and cook, covered for about 20 minutes.

With a slotted spoon, transfer the pork chops onto a plate and set aside.

In the skillet, stir in the butter until melted.

Add the heavy cream and sour cream and stir until smooth.

Stir in the cooked pork chops and cook for about 2-3 minutes or until heated completely.

Serve hot.

Nutrition:

Calories per serving: 400.

Carbohydrates: 3.6g.

Protein: 46.3g.

Fat: 21.6g.

Sugar: 0.8g.

Sodium: 820mg.

Fiber: 1.1g

South East Asian Steak Platter

Preparation Time: 15 minutes

Cooking Time: 20 minutes

Servings: 4

Ingredients:

14 oz. grass-fed sirloin steak trimmed and cut into thin strips.

Freshly ground black pepper, to taste.

2 tbsp. olive oil, divided.

1 small yellow onion, chopped.

2 garlic cloves, minced.

1 Serrano pepper seeded and chopped finely.

3 C. broccoli florets

3 tbsp. low-sodium soy sauce

2 tbsp. fresh lime juice

Directions:

Season steak with black pepper.

In a large skillet, heat 1 tbsp. of the oil over medium heat and cook the steak for about 6-8 minutes or until browned from all sides.

Transfer the steak onto a plate.

In the same skillet, heat the remaining oil and sauté onion for about 3-4 minutes.

Add the garlic and Serrano pepper and sauté for about 1 minute.

Add broccoli and stir fry for about 2-3 minutes.

Stir in cooked beef, soy sauce and lime juice and cook for about 3-4 minutes.

Serve hot.

Nutrition:

Calories per serving: 282.

Carbohydrates: 7.6g.

Protein: 33.1g.

Fat: 13.5g.

Sugar: 2.7g.

Sodium: 749mg.

Fiber: 2.3g

Pesto Flavored Steak

Preparation Time: 15 minutes

Cooking Time: 17 minutes

Servings: 4

Ingredients:

¼ C. fresh oregano, chopped.

1½ tbsp. garlic, minced.

1 tbsp. fresh lemon peel, grated.

½ tsp. red pepper flakes, crushed.

Salt and freshly ground black pepper, to taste.

1 lb. (1-inch thick) grass-fed boneless beef top sirloin steak

1 C. pesto

¼ C. feta cheese, crumbled

Directions:

Preheat the gas grill to medium heat. Lightly, grease the grill grate.

In a bowl, add the oregano, garlic, lemon peel, red pepper flakes, salt and black pepper and mix well.

Rub the garlic mixture onto the steak evenly.

Place the steak onto the grill and cook, covered for about 12-17 minutes, flipping occasionally.

Remove from the grill and place the steak onto a cutting board for about 5 minutes.

With a sharp knife, cut the steak into desired sized slices.

Divide the steak slices and pesto onto serving plates and serve with the topping of the feta cheese.

Nutrition:

Calories per serving: 226.

Carbohydrates: 6.8g.

Protein: 40.5g.

Fat: 7.6g.

Sugar: 0.7g.

Sodium: 579mg.

Fiber: 2.2g

Flawless Grilled Steak

Preparation Time: 21 minutes

Cooking Time: 10 minutes

Servings: 5

Ingredients:

½ tsp. dried thyme, crushed.

½ tsp. dried oregano, crushed.

1 tsp. red chili powder

½ tsp. ground cumin

¼ tsp. garlic powder

Salt and freshly ground black pepper, to taste.

1½ lb. grass-fed flank steak, trimmed.

¼ C. Monterrey Jack cheese, crumbled.

Directions:

In a large bowl, add the dried herbs and spices and mix well.

Add the steaks and rub with mixture generously.

Set aside for about 15-20 minutes.

Preheat the grill to medium heat. Grease the grill grate.

Place the steak onto the grill over medium coals and cook for about 17-21 minutes, flipping once halfway through.

Remove the steak from grill and place onto a cutting board for about 10 minutes before slicing.

With a sharp knife, cut the steak into desired sized slices.

Top with the cheese and serve.

Nutrition:

Calories per serving: 271.

Carbohydrates: 0.7g.

Protein: 38.3g.

Fat: 11.8g.

Sugar: 0.1g.

Sodium: 119mg.

Fiber: 0.3g

Baked Cauliflower Rice

Preparation Time: 5 minutes

Cooking Time: 20 minutes

Servings: 4

Ingredients:

- 1 big cauliflower, florets separated and riced
- 1 and ½ cups chicken stock
- 1 tablespoon olive oil
- Salt and black pepper to the taste
- ½ teaspoon turmeric powder

Directions:

1. In a pan that fits the air fryer, combine the cauliflower with the oil and the rest of the ingredients, toss, introduce in the air fryer and cook at 360 degrees F for 20 minutes.
2. Divide between plates and serve as a side dish.

Nutrition:

193 Calories

5g Fat

2g Fiber

6g Protein

Cheese Cauliflower Bake

Preparation Time: 5 minutes

Cooking Time: 20 minutes

Servings: 2

Ingredients:

- 1 cup heavy whipping cream
- 2 tablespoons basil pesto
- Salt and black pepper to the taste
- Juice of ½ lemon
- 1-pound cauliflower, florets separated
- 4 ounces cherry tomatoes, halved
- 3 tablespoons ghee, melted
- 7 ounces cheddar cheese, grated

Directions:

1. Grease a baking pan that fits the air fryer with the ghee. Add the cauliflower, lemon juice, salt, pepper, the pesto and the cream and toss gently.
2. Add the tomatoes, sprinkle the cheese on top, introduce the pan in the fryer and cook at 380 degrees F for 20 minutes. Divide between plates and serve as a side dish.

Nutrition:

200 Calories

7g Fat

2g Fiber

7g Protein

Creamy Brussels Sprouts

Preparation Time: 5 minutes

Cooking Time: 20 minutes

Servings: 4

Ingredients:

- 1-pound Brussels sprouts, trimmed and halved
- Salt and black pepper to the taste
- 2 tablespoons ghee, melted
- ½ cup coconut cream
- 2 tablespoons garlic, minced
- 1 tablespoon chives, chopped

Directions:

1. In your air fryer, mix the sprouts with the rest of the ingredients except the chives, toss well, introduce in the air fryer and cook them at 370 degrees F for 20 minutes.
2. Divide the Brussels sprouts between plates, sprinkle the chives on top, and serve as a side dish.

Nutrition:

194 Calories

6g Fat

2g Fiber

8g Protein

Mustard Broccoli and Cauliflower

Preparation Time: 5 minutes

Cooking Time: 20 minutes

Servings: 4

Ingredients:

- 15 ounces broccoli florets
- 10 ounces cauliflower florets
- 1 leek, chopped
- 2 spring onions, chopped
- Salt and black pepper to the taste
- 2 ounces butter, melted
- 2 tablespoons mustard
- 1 cup sour cream
- 5 ounces mozzarella cheese, shredded

Directions:

1. In a baking pan that fits the air fryer, add the butter and spread it well. Add the broccoli, cauliflower and the rest of the ingredients except the mozzarella and toss.

2. Sprinkle the cheese on top, introduce the pan in the air fryer and cook at 380 degrees F for 20 minutes. Divide between plates and serve as a side dish.

Nutrition:

242 Calories

13g Fat

2g Fiber

8g Protein

Mushroom Risotto

Preparation Time: 5 minutes

Cooking Time: 20 minutes

Servings: 4

Ingredients:

- 1-pound white mushrooms, sliced
- ¼ cup mozzarella, shredded
- 1 cauliflower head, florets separated and riced
- 1 cup chicken stock
- 1 tablespoon thyme, chopped
- 1 teaspoon Italian seasoning
- A pinch of salt and black pepper
- 2 tablespoons olive oil

Directions:

1. Heat up a pan that fits the air fryer with the oil over medium heat, add the cauliflower rice and the mushrooms, toss and cook for a couple of minutes.
2. Add the rest of the ingredients except the thyme, toss, put the pan in the air fryer and cook at 360 degrees F for 20 minutes.
3. Divide the risotto between plates and serve with thyme sprinkled on top

Nutrition:

204 Calories

12g Fat

3g Fiber

8g Protein

Lightning Source UK Ltd.
Milton Keynes UK
UKHW021837280621
386319UK00002B/433